Caroline Creager's
AIROBIC
BALL™
STRETCHING
WORKOUT

CAROLINE CORNING CREAGER, P.T.

EXECUTIVE PHYSICAL THERAPY INC.
BERTHOUD, COLORADO

Library of Congress Card Catalog Number: 94-90685
Creager, Caroline Corning
        The Airobic Ball™ Stretching Workout
        Creager, Caroline Corning - 1st edition

        Executive Physical Therapy, Inc.
        P.O. Box 1319
        Berthoud, CO 80513 USA
        (970) 532-2533 or 1-800-530-6878
        email: Caroline_Creager@unforgettable.com
        www.CarolineCreager.com

Printed in the United States of America
First Printing: November 1994
Second Printing: November 1998

The author has made every effort to assure that the information in this book is
accurate and current at the time of printing.The publisher and
author take no responsibility for the use of the material in this book and can
not be held responsible for any typographical or other errors found. Please
consult your physician before initiating this exercise program.
The information in this book is not intended to replace medical advice.

ISBN: 0-9641153-2-8
Library of Congress Card Catalog Number: 94-90685

Cover design by Kathy Tracy Designs, Inc.,
        Boulder, Colorado.

Book design by Alan Bernhard, Argent Associated, Inc.,
        Boulder, Colorado.

Cover Photo by Michael Cline.

Black and white Photographs by Marc Nader.

Edited by Caryl Riedel.

Cover Photo Hair and Make-up by Julie Myers and Nails by Jane Lee Mitchel.

Distributed by:
Orthopedic Physical Therapy Products
(800)367-7393 or (612)553-0452

About the Author

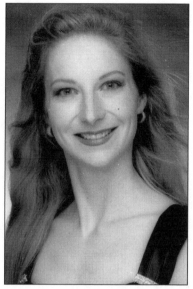

Caroline Corning Creager was born in Richmond,
Virginia, and raised in Wasilla, Alaska. She received
her degree in Physical Therapy from the University of
Montana in 1989. Caroline is a member of the American
Physical Therapy Association and the Rocky Mountain Book
Publishers Association. She is the owner of Executive
Physical Therapy, Inc. in Boulder, Colorado, and is also the
author of *The Airobic Ball™ Strengthening Workout* and
Therapeutic Exercises Using the Swiss (Airobic) Ball. She
lectures and teaches seminars throughout the United States
promoting the Airobic Ball™ stretching and strengthening
techniques and her modus operandi, "aspire to have a
healthy body, not a perfect body."

Dedication

To my husband, Robert, who needs this book more than anyone.

To my grandmothers, Hilda E. Corning and Muriel B. Reichardt, for their unwavering love and support.

To Michele Brewer Anson, for being a great friend.

To Margaret Guthrie, for her love, support, and prayers.

Acknowledgments

To Smash, Inc. Aerobic Design Wear by Jill, Greenwood
Village, Colorado, for designing my aerobic wear.

To Alan Bernhard, for his enthusiasm and creative ideas
when working with my projects.

IN MEMORY OF:

My grandfathers,

Lester Corning

&

Francis Reichardt

Table of Contents

THE AIROBIC BALL™ STRETCHING WORKOUT

MILLIONS OF PEOPLE TODAY SUFFER from muscular aches and pains. Do you have muscular aches and pains, poor posture, or lead a stressful lifestyle? Do you come home from work wondering how to rid yourself of a nagging backache, stiff shoulders, or restless wrists? If your answer is yes to any of these questions, then this book is for you.

In our present-day society, it is difficult not to become caught up in a fast paced, busy lifestyle that predisposes us to stress and muscle tension. Tension builds up in our muscles while driving, talking on the phone, or sitting at a computer terminal. These activities cause individual muscle fibers to shorten, decreasing flexibility, and increasing the likelihood of injury.

What do you need to do so you can say GOOD-BYE to aches and pains forever? Stretch! Stretching relieves stress, improves posture, decreases anxiety, and increases flexibility.

The Airobic Ball™ Stretching Workout provides more than 30 new stretching techniques to reshape your abdomen, arms, back, legs, neck, and shoulders. Unlike traditional stretching programs, the Airobic Ball™ Stretching Workout allows you to improve flexibility, balance, coordination, AND gain strength — all at the same time. More importantly, you will have fun doing these stretches.

THE BEST KEPT SECRET

ORIGINALLY, LARGE, INFLATABLE BALLS WERE USED in the 1960s by Swiss physical therapists to help children with cerebral palsy to improve their balance, reflexes, and strength. Now physical therapists and other health care professionals from around the world are teaching their clients and the general public how to break away from traditional fitness regimens and explore new strengthening, stretching, and aerobic exercises using the Airobic Ball™.

Joan Rivers reported on her late night show that the exercise ball is the workout of the "rich and famous." Liz Brody, associate editor for *Shape Magazine*, states that "We at *Shape* are willing to bet that axling balls (Airobic Balls™) become one of the next major fitness crazes—at home and in health clubs." (The Airobic Ball™ has also been coined the: Gymnic Ball, Axling Ball, and Swiss Ball.)

Mackie Shilstone, M.A., M.B.A., performance and nutrition consultant to the San Francisco Giants baseball team, St. Louis Blues hockey team, and to over 500 individual professional athletes, has been using Airobic Balls™ to improve the athletes' dynamic balance and proprioception (dynamic postural control) as well as to develop specific movement patterns that mimic game situations. Riddick Bowe, a heavyweight professional boxer, is one of the elite athletes Mackie has trained on the Airobic Ball™.

WHY IS THE AIROBIC BALL™ STRETCHING WORKOUT SO UNIQUE?

T HE AIROBIC BALL™ IS LIGHTWEIGHT and very portable. You can do this workout just about anywhere: at home, on the job, in the gym, or even in a hotel room while on a business trip or vacation.

The round, mobile surface of the Airobic Ball™ requires dormant muscles to be activated. Just sitting on the ball contracts muscles throughout your body to prevent you from rolling off the ball.

When exercising with the Airobic Ball™ your muscles contract in an eccentric manner, which promotes significant strength gains in a minimal amount of time.

The Airobic Ball™ Stretching Workout is fun, refreshing, and appropriate for all fitness levels.

Benefits of the Airobic Ball™ Stretching Workout

THE AIROBIC BALL™ BENEFITS are almost too numerous to list. All of the exercises in this book help to improve strength, posture, coordination, flexibility, balance, and endurance. The following are a few additional benefits.

- Provides a total body stretching regimen: abdomen, back, buttocks, chest, inner and outer thighs, legs, shoulders, and neck.
- Relieves muscle tension.
- Restores circulation to tense muscles.
- Helps develop body awareness.
- Improves posture and helps to align the spine.
- Reduces stress and anxiety, and reenergizes the body.
- Improves range of motion in both joints and muscles throughout the body.
- Provides a low-impact workout that does not cause undue stress on individual body parts.
- Requires inexpensive equipment and facilities.
- Provides entertainment for the entire family: adults enjoy working out on the Airobic Ball™, newborns love to be bounced to sleep on the Airobic Ball™, and children love to play with Airobic Balls™.

DETERMINING
THE APPROPRIATE
AIROBIC BALL™ SIZE

IDEALLY, IF YOU ARE SITTING ON THE BALL with your feet flat, your hips and knees should form a 90-degree angle with each other. This sitting position is called the 90-degree rule for sitting.

The following serves as a guideline for determining the appropriate Airobic Ball™ size for individuals who exercise in a sitting position:

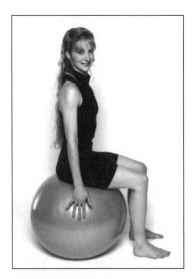

20–25 cm. ball (8-10 inches)	for non-sitting exercises requiring a small ball
30 cm. ball (14 inches)	children 1 – 2 years old
45 cm. ball (18 inches)	< 5 ft. 0 in. tall
55 cm. ball (22 inches)	5 ft. 0 in. to 5 ft. 7 in. tall
65 cm. ball (26 inches)	5 ft. 8 in. to 6 ft. 3 in. tall
75 cm. ball (30 inches)	> 6 ft. 3 in. tall

Ball size is not only determined by your height, but also by your weight and intended exercise position (sitting, lying on your back, standing, etc.). If you are 5 ft. 6 in. tall and weigh 250 pounds, I recommend the use of a 65 cm. ball. However, if you are 5 ft. 8 in. and have very short legs, you may want to try using a 55 cm. ball.

What can you do if the Airobic Ball™ you purchase is bigger in diameter than the aforementioned guidelines? The answer is, don't inflate your ball as much. For example, if you purchase a 65 cm. ball and are only 5 ft. 2 in. tall, fit the ball using the 90-degree rule in sitting. If your ball is under-inflated, the ball will not be as firm, but you will continue to reap the benefits of the Airobic Ball™.

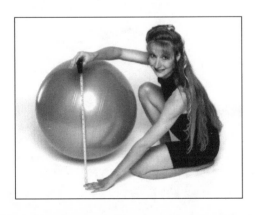

PROPER INFLATION TECHNIQUES

ALLOW THE BALL TO REACH ROOM TEMPERATURE before inflating. The Airobic Balls™ inflate to a variety of maximum diameters (i.e., 45 cm., 55 cm., etc.) and the maximum diameter is usually printed on the ball. The differing ball diameters allow inflation of balls to approximately the same firmness.

It is imperative that the recommended maximum diameter for a given ball size not be exceeded. However, underinflating the ball is perfectly acceptable.

Many methods are available for inflating the Airobic Ball™:

1. air compressor

2. hand pump

3. foot pump

4. raft pump

5. air mattress pump

6. tire pump with a trigger nozzle adapter.

The air compressor is the easiest way to inflate a ball. The air compressor forces compressed air into the ball, quickly inflating even the largest ball. Be careful not to overinflate the ball.

Hand, foot, raft, and mattress pumps are inexpensive and can be purchased for home use.

Many of these pumps can be found at a local hardware store, or from the company that sells the Airobic Ball™. Tire pumps at local gas stations can be used in conjunction with a trigger nozzle adapter to inflate the balls. Bicycle pumps are inefficient and not powerful enough to properly inflate the balls. Blowing up the balls by mouth, like the use of a bicycle pump, is also ineffective.

Every three to four months, Airobic Balls™ may require additional air. If the balls are used extensively, air may need to be added even more frequently.

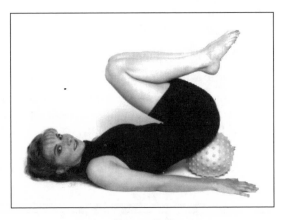

Bumpy Ball

HOW TO MEASURE THE
DIAMETER OF THE
AIROBIC BALL™

TO MEASURE THE DIAMETER OF THE BALL, use a tape measure to measure a distance of 55 centimeters (or the appropriate maximum diameter for each ball) up on a wall, beginning at floor level. Put a pencil mark on the wall at the specified height. Then, inflate the ball up to the pencil mark, using a leveled yardstick to span the distance from the mark on the wall to the center of the ball.

I have demonstrated exercises on two types of balls in this book. One is the Airobic Ball™, the large vinyl ball as mentioned previously, and the second is a small 20-cm. (8-inch) ball. The smaller ball stretches muscles at different angles and allows you to do additional exercises not practical on the larger ball.

The small bumpy ball depicted to the left prevents slippage off the ball. A child's 8-inch play ball can be used instead of the bumpy ball. You may order the bumpy ball at (800) 530-6878, or purchase a child's play ball from your local toy store.

AIROBIC BALL™
STRETCHING GUIDELINES

PROPER STRETCHING TECHNIQUES are essential to prevent muscular imbalances caused by exercise, work, or other activities of daily living. Stretching only a few muscle groups at a time may lead to muscle imbalances. A muscle imbalance occurs when one muscle such as the quadricep muscle (front thigh muscle) is more flexible than the hamstring muscle (back thigh muscle). Research, conducted by Richard Gadjosik, Ph.D., P.T., has shown that tight hamstring muscles decrease the ability of the lower back to bend forward. Muscle imbalances in hamstring and other muscle groups tend to increase the risk of injury.

WHEN TO STRETCH

The Airobic Ball™ Stretching Workout can be done at any time or any place.

- Stretch after getting out of bed and before getting into bed.

- Stretch when tension or stiffness is felt in a specific muscle.

- Stretch before and after any type of exercise.

- Stretch after driving, typing, sitting, standing, or holding the same position for an extended amount of time.
- Stretch while watching television, talking on the phone, or sitting at your desk.
- Stretch at home, at work, or at play.
- Just stretch, stretch, stretch any time of day.

Muscles should be warm before stretching. Stretching cold muscles may lead to injury. Warm up prior to stretching for 3 to 5 minutes by bouncing on the ball or walking in place while sitting on the ball.

WHEN NOT TO STRETCH

Do not stretch a muscle that has been "pulled," strained, or hurt. Wait approximately 24 to 72 hours (or until muscle soreness is gone) before initiating your stretching program. Please consult your physician or physical therapist if you have any questions as to whether you should continue with your stretching regimen.

If you have health problems, had recent surgery, or have been inactive, please consult your physician before starting this stretching program.

STRETCHING TIPS

The Airobic Ball™ Stretching Workout provides proper stretching techniques to increase muscle length, restore circulation, and promote relaxation.

To safely and effectively increase muscle length, follow the instructions given as follows:

1. Avoid bouncing.

2. Apply a slow static stretch into a level of tolerance not pain.

3. Do not hold your breath.

4. Hold stretch 15–20 seconds, unless indicated otherwise.

5. Repeat stretch to each muscle group three to five times.

6. If appropriate, repeat a stretch in opposite direction, so both sides are stretched equally.

STRETCHING PROGRAM

Stretching exercises may be done every day. You therefore have several workout options available:

1. Do all 33 Airobic Ball™ stretching exercises at each workout session every day.

2. If you find you have several favorite stretches, do those stretches every day.

3. Stretch your upper body and upper back one day and lower body and lower back the next day. A suggested workout schedule is listed below.

MONDAY & FRIDAY

Upper Body and Upper Back Workout
1. Neck Side Bends (pg. 25)
2. Neck Rotation (pg. 26)
3. Forward Neck Bend (pg. 27)

4. Backward Neck Bend (pg. 28)
5. Levator Scapulae Stretch (pg. 29)
6. Tricep Stretch (pg. 30)
7. Deltoid Stretch (pg. 31)
8. Side Stretch (pg. 32)
9. Trunk Rotation Stretch (pg. 33)
10. Chest Stretch (pg. 42)
11. Shoulder Stretch (pg. 43)
12. Shoulder Roll Stretch (pg. 44)
13. Pectoralis Stretch (pg. 45)
14. Upper Back Stretch with Small Ball (pg. 48)
15. Brachioplexus Stretch (pg. 52)
16. Standing Chest Stretch (pg. 57)

TUESDAY & SATURDAY

Lower Body and Lower Back Workout

1. Pelvic Tilt Forward and Backward (pg. 34)
2. Pelvic Circles (pg. 35)
3. Inner Thigh Stretch (pg. 36)
4. Piriformis Stretch (pg. 37)
5. Hamstring and Calf Stretch (pg. 38)
6. Hip Flexor Stretch (pg. 39)
7. Soleus Stretch (pg. 40)
8. Anterior Foot Stretch (pg. 41)
9. Knee Rolls (pg. 46)
10. Knee Rolls with Upper Body Twist (pg. 47)
11. Lower Back Stretch with Small Ball (pg. 49)
12. Side Stretch with Small Ball (pg. 50)
13. Side Stretch (pg. 51)
14. Quadricep Stretch (pg. 53)
15. Body Stretch Backward (pg. 54)
16. Body Stretch Forward (pg. 55)
17. Lower Back Stretch (pg. 56)

WEDNESDAY & SUNDAY

Favorite Stretch Workout

Do your favorite stretches, or stretch your problem areas on these days.

I have given you the option to stretch for 15 – 20 seconds on most of the stretches. You will find that some of the stretching positions will be more difficult to hold, hence stretch for 15 seconds. Others will be easier to hold for 20 seconds. When you are in a hurry, repeat stretches three times, and when you have additional time, stretch five or more times. Before deciding how many of each stretch you should do, please read LISTEN TO YOUR BODY on page 15.

LISTEN TO YOUR BODY

MANY TIMES, WHEN INDIVIDUALS BEGIN an exercise program, they forget to listen to their bodies. For example, Michael is 40 pounds overweight and has not worked out consistently for the last 10 years. He begins doing the stretch on page 32 for the first time. The book says to repeat this exercise three to five times, holding the stretch for 15 – 20 counts. Michael starts stretching to the point of pain. He remembers that in high school he was taught, "no pain, no gain," so he stretches even further. This method of stretching is INCORRECT! Stretching to the point of pain can actually cause microscopic tears to the muscle. Please review the stretching tips and listen to your body. If Michael is unable to do a specific stretch without pain, then he should not do that stretch. With time, Michael can return to the stretch he was having difficulty with, and try the stretch again following the guidelines in this book.

Design your Airobic Ball™ stretching program to meet the individualized needs of your own body. **Adapt the stretching exercise to your body. Do not adapt your body to the exercise.**

STRENGTH TRAINING

I RECOMMEND YOU AUGMENT the Airobic Ball™ Stretching Workout with a strengthening program.

Strength training will help you develop lean, mean muscle mass and burn additional calories. In order for the body to maintain muscle, it requires more oxygen and burns more calories than fat.

So the more muscle you have, the more quickly you burn calories, and the faster your metabolism works at play and at rest. Please refer to *The Airobic Ball™ Strengthening Workout* for a well-balanced strengthening program.

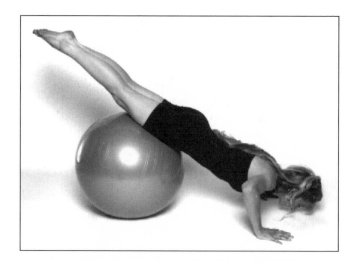

AEROBIC EXERCISE

IS STRETCHING CONSIDERED AN AEROBIC ACTIVITY? There are three requirements for an exercise to be considered aerobic:

1. The activity must use large muscles in a rhythmic manner.

2. The intensity of the workout must be between 60% – 90% of your maximal heart rate. (Please refer to: *The Airobic Ball*™ *Strengthening Workout* on HOW TO FIND YOUR TARGET HEART RATE.)

3. The duration of continuous exercise must be between 15 and 60 minutes.

No, stretching is not typically considered an aerobic activity. I recommend you augment this program with a traditional aerobic exercise program or an Airobic Ball™ cardiovascular workout. Walking, running, bicycling, in-line skating, swimming, and cross-country skiing are all excellent aerobic activities.

Regular aerobic exercise, three to four times per week, further enhances your potential to burn fat, improve stamina, and strengthen your heart and lungs.

THE FLOW SHEET

I HAVE PROVIDED A FLOW SHEET at the end of the book so you may record your progress on the number of sets and repetitions of each exercise completed, along with your daily exercise heart rate. An example is provided on page 62 to show you how to fill out the flow sheet correctly. By recording your repetitions and exercise heart rate you can see your weekly progress at a glance. If you are unfamiliar with taking your pulse to calculate your exercise heart rate, please refer to *The Airobic Ball™ Strengthening Workout.*

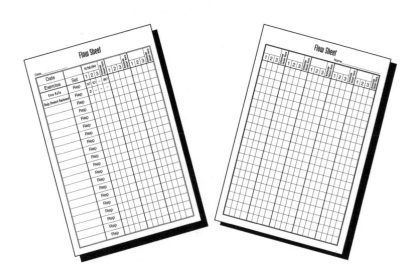

SPICE UP YOUR FOOD
AND EATING HABITS

S HAKE ALLSPICE, NUTMEG, OR CINNAMON onto your food in lieu of salt and pepper.

- Sweeten rice and other grains with apple juice while cooking.

- The recommended daily allowance of fat intake is 30% of the total calories you eat in a day.

- Simple stats on fat! An easy way to determine if a particular piece of food contains 30% of its calories from fat is to: multiply the number of fat grams found in the food by 30. If this number is less than the total number of calories in the food, it has less than 30% fat.

    For example, one bagel has approximately 160 calories and 1 gram of fat. $30 \times 1 = 30$; indicating a bagel has much less than 30% of its calories from fat.

- Fat has 9 calories per gram, carbohydrates have 4 calories per gram, and protein has 4 calories per gram.

- Cholesterol is only found in foods of animal origin.

- Try tofu and other soybean-based foods for high levels of protein and low levels of fat.

- Caffeine — to drink or not to drink? Dr. Harris Lieberman, a psychologist at M.I.T., discovered that when caffeine was consumed in the morning, mental performance improved. Hence, drink your dose of caffeine but do not overdo it. Limit caffeine intake to 300 mg./day.

- One cup of coffee contains approximately 100 mg. of caffeine. One cup of cocoa has about 10 mg., one cup of tea has 40 mg., and one dark soda pop has approximately 50 mg.

- Drink lots of water! Water helps curb the appetite and replenishes water you lose through perspiration. Drink 8 – 10 eight-ounce glasses of water a day, and an additional glass of water for each 25 pounds of extra weight you are carrying Water constitutes approximately 57% of your total body weight (Arthur Guyton, M.D., 1987). Example: A 115-pound woman's water weight would be approximately 66 pounds.

- Eat a variety of foods from the Four Food Groups:

MILK GROUP
(2 servings for adults)

One serving equals: 1 cup milk
1 oz. cheese
½ cup cottage cheese

MEAT GROUP
(2 servings)

One serving equals: 2 – 3 oz. lean meat, fish, or poultry
2 Tbs. peanut butter
½ cup beans

FRUIT AND VEGETABLE GROUP
(4 servings)

One serving equals: ½ cup juice
½ cup vegetable or fruit
1 medium apple, banana, or orange

GRAIN GROUP
(4 servings)

One serving equals: 1 slice bread
1 oz. cereal
½ cup pasta

Airobic Ball™
Stretching
Exercises

Neck Side Bends

PURPOSE:

To stretch neck muscles.

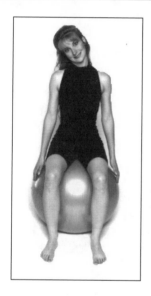

INSTRUCTION:

Sit on ball. Place hands on side of ball. Keep head/ears in line with shoulders. Bend head sideways toward shoulder. Repeat on opposite side.

HOLD:

15 – 20 seconds

REPEAT:

3 – 5 times

Neck Rotation

PURPOSE:
To stretch neck muscles.

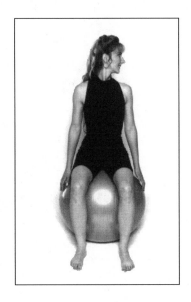

INSTRUCTION:

Sit on ball. Place hands on side of ball. Rotate head slowly to the right and look over shoulder. Repeat to the left.

HOLD:

15 – 20 seconds

REPEAT:

3 – 5 times

Forward Neck Bend

PURPOSE:
To stretch back of neck muscles.

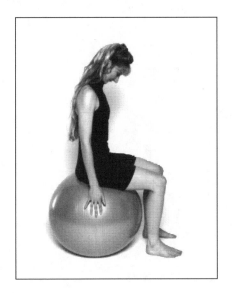

INSTRUCTION:

Sit on ball. Place hands on side of ball. Slowly lower head to chest.

HOLD:

15 – 20 seconds

REPEAT:

3 – 5 times

Backward Neck Bend

PURPOSE:

To stretch front of neck muscles.

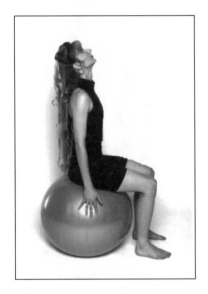

INSTRUCTION:

Sit on ball. Place hands on side of ball. Slowly lower head toward back.

HOLD:

15 – 20 seconds

REPEAT:

3 – 5 times

Levator Scapulae Stretch

PURPOSE:
To stretch back of neck muscles.

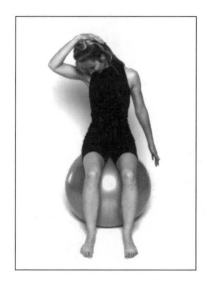

INSTRUCTION:

Sit on ball. Place right hand behind head. Extend left arm slightly behind back and reach for floor. Bend neck forward and look down at right knee. Repeat with left hand and right arm.

HOLD:

15 – 20 seconds

REPEAT:

3 – 5 times

Tricep Stretch

PURPOSE:
To stretch back of arm muscles.

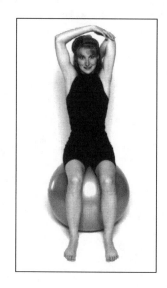

INSTRUCTION:

Sit on ball. Bend left elbow and place behind head. Place right hand on left elbow and press down lightly. Repeat with opposite arm.

HOLD:

15 – 20 seconds

REPEAT:

3 – 5 times

Deltoid Stretch

PURPOSE:
To stretch shoulder muscles.

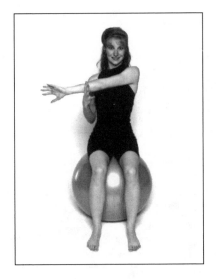

INSTRUCTION:

Sit on ball. Raise left arm to shoulder height, in front of body. Place right hand on left upper arm and pull left arm across body. Repeat with opposite arm.

HOLD:

15 – 20 seconds

REPEAT:

3 – 5 times

Side Stretch

PURPOSE:
To stretch side of trunk muscles.

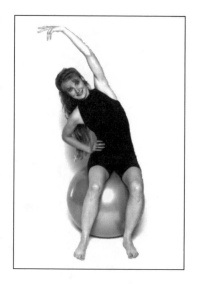

INSTRUCTION:

Sit on ball. Place right hand on hip. Raise left arm overhead.
Bend at waist to right side and shift weight to left hip.
Repeat to opposite side.

HOLD:

15 – 20 seconds

REPEAT:

3 – 5 times

Trunk Rotation Stretch

PURPOSE:
To stretch shoulder and torso muscles.

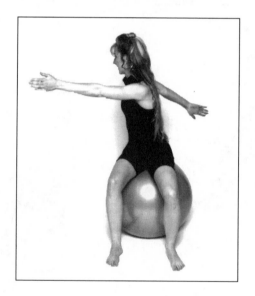

INSTRUCTION:

Sit on ball. Extend arms and rotate. Turn head with upper body. Repeat in opposite direction.

HOLD:

15 – 20 seconds

REPEAT:

3 – 5 times

PRECAUTION:
Keep lower body
stationary.

Pelvic Tilt Forward and Backward

PURPOSE:
To stretch abdominal and back muscles.

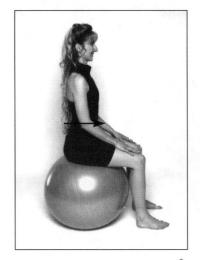
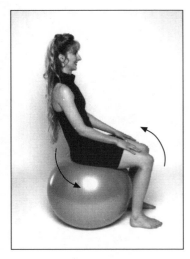

INSTRUCTION:
Sit on ball. Roll ball backward as hips roll forward. Slightly arch back. Return to starting position. Roll ball forward as hips roll backward. Return to starting position.

HOLD:
3 – 5 seconds

REPEAT:
8 – 12 times

Pelvic Circles

PURPOSE:
To stretch back and hip muscles.

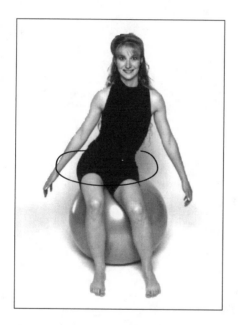

INSTRUCTION:

Sit on ball. Begin drawing a circle, initiating movement from hips. Rotate hips clockwise, then rotate hips counter-clockwise.

REPEAT:

8 – 12 times

Inner Thigh Stretch

PURPOSE:
To stretch inner thigh muscles.

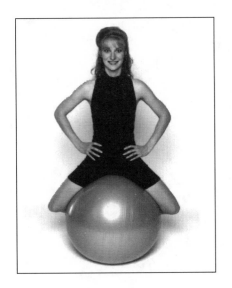

INSTRUCTION:
Sit on ball. Place hands on hips. Slide one knee around to side of ball. Slide other knee around to opposite side of ball. Toes touch floor behind ball.

HOLD:
15 – 20 seconds

REPEAT:
3 – 5 times

Piriformis Stretch

PURPOSE:
To stretch buttock muscles.

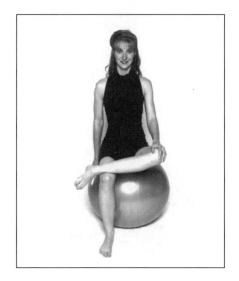

INSTRUCTION:

Sit on ball. Place right hand on side of ball. Bend left knee and place heel on right knee. Place left hand on left knee and lightly press knee toward floor. Repeat with opposite leg.

HOLD:

15 – 20 seconds

REPEAT:

3 – 5 times

PRECAUTION:

For added stability, hold onto couch with right hand. Be careful!

Hamstring and Calf Stretch

PURPOSE:
To stretch back of thigh and calf muscles.

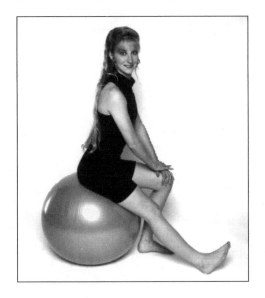

INSTRUCTION:

Sit on ball. Lean forward at waist. Place hands on bent knee. Straighten opposite leg. Pull toes up toward ceiling. Repeat with opposite side.

HOLD:

15 – 20 seconds

REPEAT:

3 – 5 times

Hip Flexor Stretch

PURPOSE:
To stretch hip muscles.

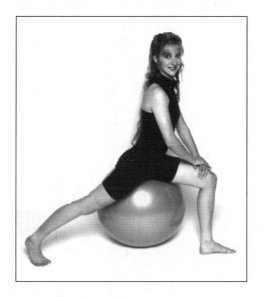

INSTRUCTION:

Sit on ball. Slide one leg behind ball. Straighten back leg. Keep front leg bent. Place hands on bent knee. Repeat with opposite side.

HOLD:

15 – 20 seconds

REPEAT:

3 – 5 times

Soleus Stretch

PURPOSE:

To stretch shin muscles.

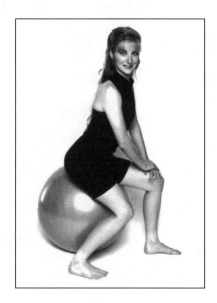

INSTRUCTION:

Sit on ball. Move one foot back beside ball. Lean forward at waist. Repeat with opposite side.

HOLD:

15 – 20 seconds

REPEAT:

3 – 5 times

Anterior Foot Stretch

PURPOSE:
To stretch front of foot muscles.

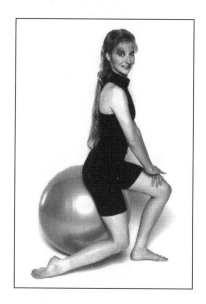

INSTRUCTION:

Sit on ball. Point toe and move foot back beside ball so top of foot faces downward. Repeat with opposite side.

HOLD:

15 – 20 seconds

REPEAT:

3 – 5 times

Chest Stretch

PURPOSE:
To stretch chest muscles.

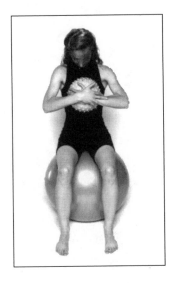

INSTRUCTION:
Sit on ball. Place small ball between chest and hands. Inhale and slowly lower head toward chest. Exhale as hands press ball into chest.

HOLD:
15 – 20 seconds

REPEAT:
3 – 5 times

Shoulder Stretch

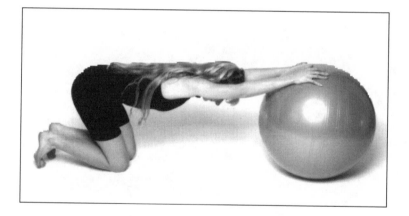

INSTRUCTION:

Kneel. Lean forward and roll ball away from body. Keep hands on ball and arms out straight.

HOLD:

15 – 20 seconds

REPEAT:

3 – 5 times

Shoulder Roll Stretch

PURPOSE:

To stretch shoulder and upper back muscles.

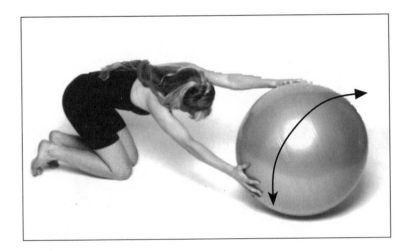

INSTRUCTION:

Kneel. Lean forward and roll ball away from body. Keep hands on ball and arms out straight. Roll ball from side to side.

HOLD:

3 – 5 seconds

REPEAT:

5 – 10 times

Pectoralis Stretch

PURPOSE:
To stretch chest muscles.

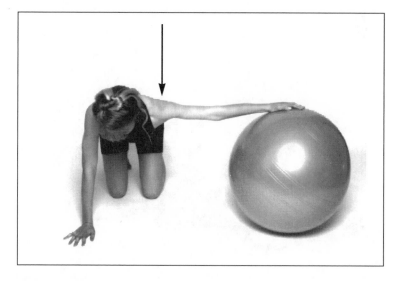

INSTRUCTION:

Kneel. Place one hand on floor and one hand on ball. Roll ball out to side of body. Lightly press shoulder toward floor. Repeat with opposite arm.

HOLD:

15 – 20 seconds

REPEAT:

3 – 5 times

Knee Rolls

PURPOSE:
To stretch torso muscles.

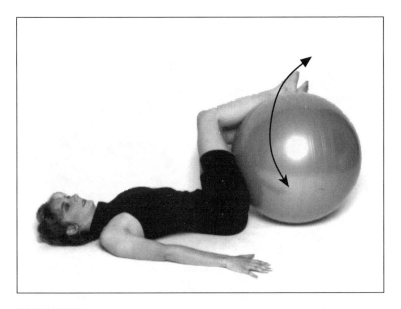

INSTRUCTION:

Lie on back with legs on ball. Roll ball from side to side using knees.

HOLD:

3 seconds

REPEAT:

5 – 10 times

Knee Rolls with Upper Body Twist

PURPOSE:
To stretch torso muscles.

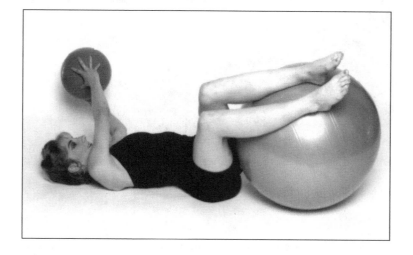

INSTRUCTION:
Lie on back with legs on ball. Place a small ball between hands and raise arms. Move arms to left and knees to right. Repeat in opposite direction.

HOLD:
5 seconds

REPEAT:
5 – 10 times

Upper Back Stretch with Small Ball

PURPOSE:
To stretch upper back muscles.

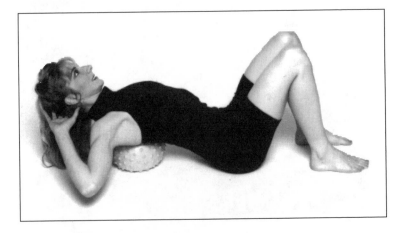

INSTRUCTION:

Lie on side. Place ball next to upper back. Roll onto ball.
Inhale. Place unclasped hands behind head. Exhale. Gently
lower head and shoulders until light resistance is felt.

HOLD:

15 – 20 seconds

REPEAT:

3 – 5 times

PRECAUTION:
Do not arch back
excessively.

ALTERNATIVE:

Place ball at different levels of upper back.

Lower Back Stretch with Small Ball

PURPOSE:
To stretch lower back muscles.

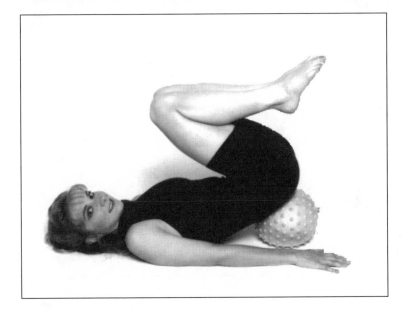

INSTRUCTION:
Lie on back. Bend knees toward chest. Place small ball under buttocks.

HOLD:
15 – 20 seconds

REPEAT:
3 – 5 times

Side Stretch with Small Ball

PURPOSE:

To stretch torso muscles.

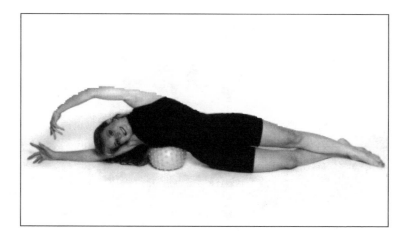

INSTRUCTION:

Lie on ball. Place small ball under torso. Raise arms
overhead. Repeat with opposite side.

HOLD:

15 – 20 seconds

REPEAT:

3 – 5 times

Side Stretch

PURPOSE:

To stretch torso muscles.

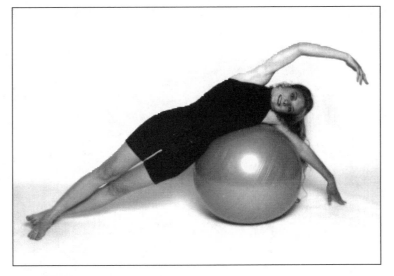

INSTRUCTION:

Kneel. Place ball alongside body. Stretch over ball with one arm overhead. Straighten top leg, then bottom leg. Repeat with opposite side.

HOLD:

15 – 20 seconds

REPEAT:

3 – 5 times

Brachioplexus Stretch

PURPOSE:
To stretch shoulder and chest muscles.

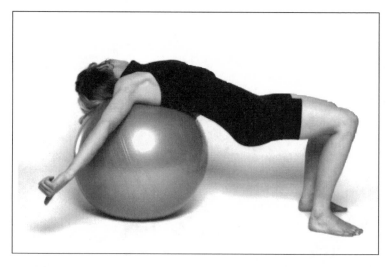

INSTRUCTION:

Sit on ball. Walk feet out so head and shoulders are resting on ball. Stretch one arm overhead and rotate hand so palm is facing ceiling and thumb is pointing toward floor. Rotate head in opposite direction. Repeat with opposite arm.

HOLD:

15 – 20 seconds

REPEAT:

3 – 5 times

Quadricep Stretch

PURPOSE:
To stretch front of thigh muscles.

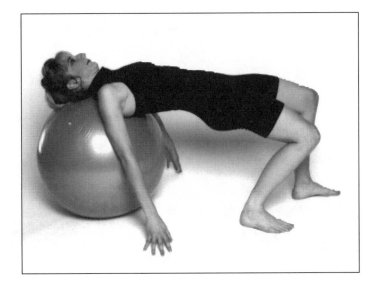

INSTRUCTION:

Sit on ball. Walk feet out so head and shoulders rest on ball. Slide one heel back toward head. Repeat with opposite side.

HOLD:

15 – 20 seconds

REPEAT:

3 – 5 times

PRECAUTION:
Do not let buttocks sag.

Body Stretch Backward

PURPOSE:

To stretch abdominal, arm, leg, back, and neck muscles.

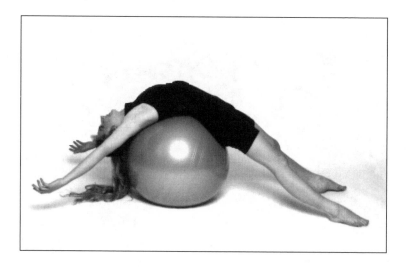

INSTRUCTION:

Sit on ball. Walk legs out away from ball so head and shoulders rest on ball. Raise arms overhead and straighten legs out.

HOLD:

15 – 20 seconds

REPEAT:

3 – 5 times

122222222

2221

221

122

Body Stretch Forward

PURPOSE:
To stretch back and neck muscles.

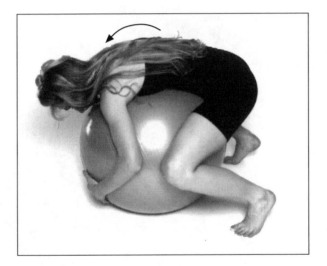

INSTRUCTION:
Kneel. Lie with abdomen on ball. Bend knees and place on each side of ball. Bend elbows and relax head down. Lean forward over ball.

HOLD:
15–20 seconds

REPEAT:
3–5 times

Lower Back Stretch

PURPOSE:

To stretch lower back muscles.

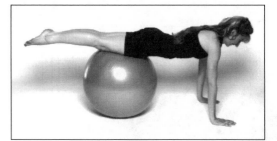

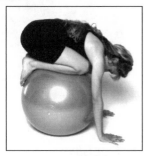

INSTRUCTION:

Kneel. Lie with abdomen on ball. Walk arms out until thighs are on ball. Bring knees to chest until body is in a tuck position.

HOLD:

15 – 20 seconds

REPEAT:

3 – 5 times

Standing Chest Stretch

PURPOSE:
To stretch chest muscles.

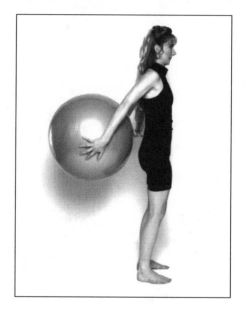

INSTRUCTION:

Stand. Grasp ball behind back. Lift ball up toward ceiling.

HOLD:

15 – 20 seconds

REPEAT:

3 – 5 times

PRECAUTION:

Do not lean forward
with body.

REFERENCES

Anderson, Bob. *Stretching.* Bolinas: Shelter Publications, 1991.

American Heart Association Pamphlet, 1994.

Brody, Liz. "Axling: A New Spin on Fitness," *Shape Magazine*, April 1993: pp. 80 – 93.

Creager, Caroline Corning. *The Airobic Ball™ Strengthening Workout.* Boulder: Executive Physical Therapy, 1994.

Creager, Caroline Corning. *Therapeutic Exercises Using the Swiss Ball.* Boulder: Executive Physical Therapy, 1994.

Gadjosik, Richard, et al. "Influence of Hamstring Length on the Standing Position and Flexion Range of Motion of the Pelvic Angle, Lumbar Angle, and Thoracic Angle." *Journal of Orthopaedic and Sports Physical Therapy*, 20 (4): 213–219, 1994.

Guidelines for Exercise Testing and Prescription. Philadelphia; Lea & Febiger, 1986.

Guyton, Arthur. *Human Physiology and Mechanism of Disease.* Philadelphia: W.B. Saunders, 1987.

Keehan, Jane. "Eccentric Exercise—Delayed Muscle Soreness vs. Training Benefits." *Physical Therapy Forum*, May 13, 1992.

Lockette, Kevin, & Keyes, Ann. *Conditioning with Physical Disabilities.* Champaign: Human Kinetics, 1994.

Pollock, Michael et al. *Exercise in Health and Disease.* Philadelphia: W. B. Saunders Company, 1984.

Rocabado, Mariano, & Antoniotti, Terri. *Exercise and Total Well Being For Vertebral and Craniomandibular Disorders.* Santiago: IFORC Publications, 1990.

Smith, Craig. "The Warm-up Procedure: To Stretch or Not to Stretch: A Brief Review." *Journal of Orthopaedic and Sports Physical Therapy,* 19(1): 1217, 1994.

Suggested Reading

 Creager, Caroline Corning. *The Airobic Ball™ Strengthening Workout*, Berthoud, CO: Executive Physical Therapy Inc., 1994.

 Creager, Caroline Corning. *Therapeutic Exercises Using the Swiss Ball*, Berthoud, CO: Executive Physical Therapy Inc., 1994.

 Creager, Caroline Corning. *Therapeutic Exercises Using Foam Rollers*, Berthoud, CO: Executive Physical Therapy Inc., 1996.

 Creager, Caroline Corning. *Therapeutic Exercises Using Resistive Bands*, Berthoud, CO: Executive Physical Therapy Inc., 1998.

For more information on ordering these books, please call:

United States/Canada
O.P.T.P.: (800) 367-7393 or (612) 553-0452

Australia/New Zealand
Sport Speed: 61 (02) 6772 7433

United Kingdom
Osteopathic Supplies Limited: 01432 263939

Flow Sheet

Date_____

Date		11/16/94			EXERCISE HEART RATE				EXERCISE HEART RATE			
Exercise	Set	1	2	3		1	2	3		1	2	3
Knee Rolls	Rep	10	10	–	90							
Body Stretch Backward	Rep	3	–	–	–							
	Rep											
	Rep											
	Rep											
	Rep											
	Rep											
	Rep											
	Rep											
	Rep											
	Rep											
	Rep											
	Rep											
	Rep											
	Rep											
	Rep											
	Rep											
	Rep											
	Rep											
	Rep											
	Rep											